Beating Heart Disease:

A Holistic Approach to Cardiovascular Health

Jeffrey E. Gardner

TABLE OF CONTENTS

Introduction

Why Cardiovascular Health Matters

Jack was a youthful, bright, and industrious guy who put in long hours at the workplace and frequently ate fast food on the run. He didn't have time for exercising or taking care of his health. He didn't worry much about his cardiovascular health, believing that he was young and healthy.

One day, while at work, Jack started to feel a searing discomfort in his chest. He attempted to ignore it, believing it was only a muscular spasm, but the agony just became worse. Soon, Jack was having problems breathing and his employees took him to the hospital.

The physicians instantly discovered that Jack was experiencing a heart attack. They fought to save his life, but the harm had already been done. Jack was left with irreversible cardiac damage and had to endure many operations to restore his heart.

This encounter was a wake-up call for Jack. He recognized that he had been taking his health for granted and needed to make some substantial adjustments. He started to eat a nutritious diet, rich in fruits, vegetables, and lean meats. He began to exercise consistently, even if it was only a short stroll each day.

Over time, Jack started to realize the advantages of these modifications. He had more energy, felt less worried, and his general health improved. He also found that taking care of his cardiovascular health wasn't only about avoiding heart attacks, but it also helped him avoid other health conditions including stroke, diabetes, and high blood pressure.

Jack's tale is a reminder that cardiovascular health matters. Our heart is the most vital muscle in our body and it has to be taken care of. Cardiovascular disease is the largest cause of mortality globally, yet it's also completely avoidable.

There are various things we may take to enhance our cardiovascular health. Eating a good diet, exercising frequently, and controlling stress are all crucial. We should also avoid smoking and restrict our alcohol usage.

Regular check-ups with our physicians are also vital. They may help us discover any possible cardiovascular concerns early on and offer us the tools and knowledge we need to take care of our hearts.

In the end, taking care of our cardiovascular health isn't only about avoiding heart attacks or other ailments, but it's about living a longer, better life. Like Jack, we should all commit to taking care of our hearts and making our health a high priority.

What Exactly Is Heart Disease?

Heart disease, often known as cardiovascular disease, is a collection of disorders that affect the heart and blood arteries. It is one of the top causes of mortality globally, accounting for nearly 17 million fatalities each year.

There are various forms of cardiac disease, including:

Coronary artery disease: This happens when the arteries that provide blood to the heart become constricted or clogged, limiting blood flow to the heart muscle.

Heart failure: This occurs when the heart can't pump enough blood to fulfill the body's demands.

Arrhythmias: Refers to abnormal cardiac rhythms, which may be life-threatening in certain situations.

Heart valve disease: This occurs when the valves that control blood flow in the heart don't work correctly.

Cardiomyopathy: Refers to illnesses of the heart muscle.

Aortic aneurysm: Occurs when the aorta (the primary artery that delivers blood from the heart to the rest of the body) gets swollen.

No matter the level of your heart presently, don't be silent about it. Do something quickly before it stops you forever.

Various risk factors might contribute to the development of heart disease. These include:

High blood pressure: When blood pressure is continuously high, it may damage the blood vessels and raise the risk of heart disease.

High cholesterol: High levels of cholesterol in the blood may contribute to the formation of plaque in the arteries, raising the risk of coronary heart disease.

Smoking: Smoking destroys the blood vessels and raises the risk of heart disease.

Diabetes: People with diabetes are at a higher risk of getting heart disease.

Obesity: Being overweight or obese may raise the chance of having heart disease.

Family history of heart disease: If someone in your family has had heart disease, you may be at an elevated risk.

Age: The risk of heart disease grows as we become older.

Preventing heart disease entails adopting good lifestyle choices. This might include:

Eating a nutritious diet: A diet that is low in saturated and trans fats, cholesterol, salt, and added sweets may help minimize the risk of heart disease.

Exercising regularly: Aim for at least 30 minutes of moderate-intensity activity most days of the week.

Maintaining a healthy weight: Being overweight or obese might raise the risk of heart disease.

Managing stress: Chronic stress may contribute to the development of heart disease.

Not smoking or using tobacco products: Smoking destroys the blood vessels and raises the risk of heart disease.

Limiting alcohol intake: Excessive alcohol drinking may raise the risk of heart disease.

Managing underlying health conditions: Conditions including high blood pressure, high cholesterol, and diabetes may raise the risk of heart disease. Managing these circumstances may help lower the risk.

If you have risk factors for heart disease or are experiencing symptoms like chest discomfort, shortness of breath, or exhaustion, it's crucial to speak to your doctor. They can help you evaluate your risk and design a strategy to help avoid heart disease or manage your symptoms.

A Holistic Approach

A holistic approach to heart disease is significant because it addresses all elements of a person's health and well-being, rather than only treating the symptoms of heart disease. By adopting a complete approach to heart health, a holistic approach may promote overall health and lower the risk of heart disease.

Some particular advantages of a holistic approach to heart disease include:

Reducing Risk Variables: A holistic approach to heart disease focuses on identifying and resolving the core causes of heart disease, such as poor nutrition, lack of exercise, stress, and environmental variables. By addressing these risk factors, a comprehensive approach may help minimize the risk of heart disease.

Improving Heart Health: A holistic approach to heart disease includes lifestyle adjustments, such as good food, frequent exercise, and stress reduction approaches. These lifestyle alterations may assist improve heart health, such as decreasing blood pressure, reducing inflammation, and improving cholesterol levels.

Addressing Emotional and Mental Health: A holistic approach to heart disease takes into consideration the emotional and mental health of a person since these aspects might contribute to the development of heart disease. By treating emotional and mental health difficulties, such as sadness or anxiety, a holistic approach may enhance overall health and minimize the risk of heart disease.

Providing tailored treatment: A holistic approach to heart disease entails designing a tailored treatment plan that takes into consideration an individual's unique requirements and preferences. By personalizing treatment to the individual, a holistic approach may deliver more effective and efficient care.

Complementing Conventional Treatment: A holistic approach to heart disease may be utilized in combination with conventional medical therapies, such as medication or surgery. By embracing complementary and alternative treatments, such as acupuncture or herbal therapy, a holistic approach may give a more thorough and successful treatment strategy.

In conclusion, heart disease is a dangerous disorder that affects millions of individuals globally. By adopting good lifestyle choices and controlling underlying health concerns, we may lower our chance of developing heart disease and live longer healthier lives.

This book promises to give revelatory insights into cardiovascular diseases, types, causes, symptoms, treatments, and how to prevent them completely.

Part I: The Fundamentals of Cardiovascular Health

Chapter One:

The Role of Nutrition in Heart Health

The impact of diet on heart health is crucial and cannot be emphasized. Heart disease is one of the main causes of mortality globally, and the frequency of the condition is only growing. While genetics and lifestyle variables such as smoking and lack of exercise have a part, diet is a significant element in the development and prevention of heart disease.

Dietary variables such as saturated and trans fats, high salt, and added sugar may raise the risk of heart disease. On the other hand, a diet rich in fruits, vegetables, whole grains, and healthy fats may minimize the risk. The goal is to have a balanced diet that delivers all the required elements for good heart health.

One of the most critical components of a heart-healthy diet is the kind of fats ingested. Saturated and trans fats found in animal products, fried meals, and baked goods may elevate cholesterol levels and increase the risk of heart disease. On the other side, unsaturated fats, such as those found in nuts, seeds, and fish, may decrease cholesterol levels and lessen the risk of heart disease. Consuming foods rich in unsaturated fats, such as avocados, olive oil, and fatty seafood, may have a substantial influence on heart health.

Another vital component for heart health is fiber. Fiber is found in fruits, vegetables, and whole grains and is crucial for maintaining healthy cholesterol levels and decreasing the risk of heart disease. Soluble fiber, in particular, has been demonstrated to reduce LDL cholesterol levels, popularly known as "bad" cholesterol. Foods rich in soluble fiber include oatmeal, beans, and apples.

In addition to these basic nutrients, several foods provide nutrients that are especially advantageous for heart health. For example, dark chocolate has flavonoids that may help decrease blood pressure, and almonds include vitamin E, which helps lessen the risk of heart disease. Eating a range of full, nutrient-dense meals is the greatest approach to guarantee that you're receiving all the required nutrients for optimum heart health.

It's not only about what you eat but also about what you don't consume. Consuming excessive quantities of salt may elevate blood pressure, which is a risk factor for heart disease. Sodium is typically present in processed meals, canned foods, and fast food. To minimize salt consumption, it's vital to pick fresh, whole foods and to read product labels carefully. The American Heart Association advises taking no more than 2,300 milligrams of sodium per day, which is roughly a teaspoon of salt.

In addition to a balanced diet, keeping a healthy weight, participating in regular physical exercise, avoiding smoking, and managing stress are all critical for heart health. These lifestyle variables may work in unison with an appropriate diet to prevent and control heart disease.

The Heart-Healthy Diet

A heart-healthy diet is rich in nutrients and low in saturated and trans fats, added sweets, and salt. Such a diet may help to minimize the risk of heart disease, an illness that affects millions of people worldwide. We will review the fundamentals of a heart-healthy diet, the foods that should be included, and those that should be restricted.

Principles of a Heart-Healthy Diet:

The fundamentals of a heart-healthy diet include having a balanced meal that is rich in nutrients, low in saturated and trans fats, and devoid of added sweets and excessive quantities of salt. The diet should consist of entire foods that are minimally processed and as near to their original condition as possible.

The diet should also contain a variety of fruits, vegetables, whole grains, lean meats, and healthy fats. Whole grains such as brown rice, quinoa, and whole wheat bread deliver fiber, vitamins, and minerals that are vital for heart health. Lean proteins such as chicken, fish, legumes, and tofu are good sources of protein without the extra saturated fats found in red meat.

Fruits and vegetables are rich in vitamins, minerals, and antioxidants that assist to decrease inflammation and prevent the accumulation of plaque in the arteries. Healthy fats such as those found in nuts, seeds, avocado, and olive oil are necessary for heart health and may help to decrease cholesterol levels.

Foods to Include:
Fruits and vegetables should make up a large percentage of a heart-healthy diet. These meals are low in calories and rich in nutrients and fiber. They also include antioxidants that assist

to decrease inflammation and prevent the formation of plaque in the arteries. Some of the greatest fruits and vegetables for heart health include:

Berries: Blueberries, strawberries, raspberries, and blackberries are all rich in antioxidants and fiber.
Leafy Greens: Spinach, kale, and collard greens are good sources of vitamins A, C, and K plus minerals such as calcium and magnesium.

Cruciferous Vegetables: Broccoli, cauliflower, and Brussels sprouts contain antioxidants that assist to decrease inflammation and prevent the accumulation of plaque in the arteries.

Tomatoes: Tomatoes contain lycopene, an antioxidant that has been associated with a lower risk of heart disease.

Citrus Fruits: Oranges, lemons, and grapefruits are all high in vitamin C, which has been associated with a lower risk of heart disease.

Whole grains should also be included in a heart-healthy diet. These foods are high in fiber, which helps to decrease cholesterol levels and lessen the risk of heart disease. Some of the greatest whole grains for heart health include:

Oats: Oats include a form of soluble fiber called beta-glucan, which has been demonstrated to reduce LDL cholesterol levels.
Brown Rice: Brown rice is a complete grain that is high in fiber and vitamins and minerals such as magnesium and selenium.

Quinoa: Quinoa is a protein-dense whole grain that is also high in fiber, vitamins, and minerals.
Healthy fats should also be included in a heart-healthy diet. These fats may assist to decrease cholesterol levels and lessen the risk of heart disease. Some of the greatest sources of healthy fats include:

Nuts and Seeds: Almonds, walnuts, chia seeds, and flaxseeds are all wonderful sources of healthful fats.

Avocado: Avocado is a great source of monounsaturated fats, which may assist to decrease cholesterol levels.

Olive Oil: Olive oil is an excellent source of monounsaturated fats and has been linked to a lower risk of heart disease.

Foods to Limit:
Saturated and trans fats, added sweets, and excessive quantities of salt should be restricted in a heart-healthy diet. These saturated and trans fats added sugars, and excessive quantities of salt should be restricted in a heart-healthy diet. These foods have been related to an elevated risk of heart disease and should be taken in moderation. Some of the items that should be restricted in a heart-healthy diet include:

Red Meat: Red meat is heavy in saturated fats, which may elevate cholesterol levels and increase the risk of heart disease.

Processed Meats: Processed meats such as bacon, sausage, and deli meats are rich in salt and may raise the risk of heart disease.

Fried meals: Fried meals are rich in trans fats, which may elevate cholesterol levels and increase the risk of heart disease.

Sugary beverages: Sugary beverages such as soda and sports drinks are rich in added sugars, which may raise the risk of heart disease.

rich-salt Foods: Foods that are rich in salt, such as canned soups, frozen dinners, and fast food, may elevate blood pressure and increase the risk of heart disease.

The Importance of Nutrient Density

While numerous variables contribute to the development of heart disease, including genetics, lifestyle choices, and environmental factors, one critical element that is frequently neglected is nutritional density.

Nutrient density refers to the number of nutrients per calorie in a diet or meal. In other words, it is a measure of how much nutrition you are receiving for the quantity of energy (calories) you are ingesting. Foods that are rich in nutritional density contain a broad variety of critical vitamins, minerals, and other nutrients that are necessary for maintaining good health and avoiding chronic conditions like heart disease.

In contrast, foods that are poor in nutrient density are generally rich in calories but give a little nutritious benefit. These foods may lead to weight gain, vitamin deficiencies, and other health concerns that raise the risk of heart disease.

Many chronic illnesses are connected to inadequate nutrition, including diabetes, cancer, and respiratory ailments. By selecting nutrient-dense meals, you may minimize your chance of these other health concerns, which can in turn lessen your risk of heart disease.

The Importance of Nutrient Density in Preventing or Treating Heart Disease

Nutrient-dense meals give crucial vitamins and minerals that are required for heart health.

Many vitamins and minerals are crucial for supporting a healthy heart, including magnesium, potassium, calcium, vitamin D, and folate. These minerals assist to control blood pressure, avoid blood clots, and support healthy blood flow, among other advantages. Nutrient-dense meals including fruits, vegetables, whole grains, and lean meats are all rich providers of these vital elements.

Nutrient-dense meals are frequently rich in fiber, which is crucial for heart health.

Fiber is a form of carbohydrate that is not broken down by the body. Instead, it travels through the digestive system largely intact, giving a variety of health advantages. One of the primary advantages of fiber is that it helps to decrease cholesterol levels, which may lessen the risk of heart disease. Fiber also helps to control blood sugar levels, which is vital for avoiding diabetes, another risk factor for heart disease. Nutrient-dense foods including fruits, vegetables, whole grains, and legumes are all rich sources of fiber.

Nutrient-dense diets may assist to lower inflammation, which is a key factor in heart disease.
Inflammation is a normal reaction to injury or illness, but persistent inflammation may lead to several health concerns, including heart disease. Certain nutrients, including omega-3 fatty acids, antioxidants, and phytochemicals, have been demonstrated to have anti-inflammatory properties. Nutrient-dense foods including fatty fish, nuts, berries, and leafy greens are all rich providers of these anti-inflammatory elements.

Nutrient-dense meals may assist you to maintain a healthy weight, which is vital for heart health.
Maintaining a healthy weight is a key aspect of avoiding heart disease. Obesity and overweight are both substantial risk factors for heart

disease, since they may lead to high blood pressure, high cholesterol, and other health concerns. Nutrient-dense meals are frequently low in calories but rich in nutrients, which may assist to increase fullness and lessen cravings for high-calorie, low-nutrient foods.

Nutrient-dense diets may assist to enhance overall health, lowering the risk of various health conditions that can lead to heart disease.

Whole Foods
Whole foods are foods that are little processed and have no extra substances. These foods are in their original condition and have not been drained of their nutrients or changed in any manner. Examples of entire foods include fruits, vegetables, whole grains, nuts, seeds, and legumes.

Whole foods are often unprocessed or slightly refined, which indicates that they still include all of their natural nutrients, fiber, and other beneficial ingredients. For example, whole grains have bran, germ, and endosperm, which give a spectrum of vitamins, minerals, and fiber. In contrast, refined grains have been stripped of the bran and germ, which eliminates many of the minerals and fiber.

Whole foods are also frequently devoid of additives, preservatives, and artificial tastes and colors, which may have harmful impacts on health. By eating whole foods, you are supplying your body with the critical nutrients it needs to operate correctly and support overall health and well-being.

In recent years, the eating of whole foods has grown more popular as people become more aware of the health advantages of a whole food diet. Whole foods may be purchased at farmers' markets, health food shops, and select grocery stores, and can be included in a range of meals and snacks.

Overall, whole foods are a healthy and enjoyable method to nourish your body and support excellent health. By selecting whole foods over processed or refined meals, you may promote good health and well-being.

Benefits of including whole foods in your diet

Nutrient density: Whole foods are rich in critical vitamins, minerals, and other nutrients that are needed for optimal health. These nutrients are typically lost or decreased in processed meals. For example, whole grains are rich in fiber, B vitamins, and minerals like magnesium and selenium, while fruits and vegetables are high in vitamin C, vitamin A, and other antioxidants.

Digestive health: Whole foods are high in fiber, which helps to promote healthy digestion and avoid constipation. Fiber also feeds the good bacteria in the gut, which may enhance gut health and boost general health and immunity.

Weight control: Whole foods are frequently fewer in calories and richer in fiber than processed meals, which may aid with weight management. Fiber also enhances feelings of fullness and may reduce overeating, which can assist to maintain a healthy weight.

Blood sugar control: Whole foods are frequently low in added sugars and processed carbs, which may assist to manage blood sugar levels and avoid insulin resistance. This may be especially essential for persons with diabetes or those at risk of acquiring diabetes.

Heart health: Whole foods are rich in heart-friendly elements including fiber, vitamins, minerals, and healthy fats. Consuming a diet rich in whole foods has been associated with a decreased risk of heart disease, stroke, and other cardiovascular disorders.

Improved mood and energy levels: Whole meals provide critical nutrients that help promote excellent mental health and energy levels. For example, omega-3 fatty acids found in fatty fish and nuts have been proven to promote mood, while B vitamins found in whole grains help support energy levels and cognitive function.

Sustainable Strategies for Healthy Eating

Eating a balanced diet is essential for overall health and avoiding chronic illnesses, but it may be difficult to maintain healthy eating habits over time. Fortunately, there are many tactics you may use to make healthy eating both sustainable and pleasant.

schedule Ahead: One of the most important methods for sustaining healthy eating is to schedule your meals ahead of time. This entails planning your meals for the week, creating a grocery list, and doing your grocery shopping ahead of time. When hunger hits, having nutritious meals on hand will help you avoid the urge to go for bad choices.

Make minor adjustments: Making minor adjustments is another crucial method for making healthy eating sustainable. Trying to fully revamp your diet all at once might be daunting and difficult to maintain in the long run. Instead, begin by making tiny modifications to your diet, such as including extra vegetables in your meals or substituting healthier snacks for bad ones. These tiny modifications may build up over time and contribute to a better overall diet.

Focus on Whole Foods: Focusing on whole foods is one of the most significant methods for making healthy eating sustainably. Whole foods are those that have been lightly processed and do not include any extra ingredients. These foods are in their original condition, with no nutrients removed or manipulated in any manner. Fruits, vegetables, whole grains, nuts, seeds, and legumes are examples of whole foods. Focusing on whole meals may help your body get the critical nutrients it needs to be healthy and avoid chronic illnesses.

Cook at Home: Cooking at home as often as possible is another crucial method for making healthy eating sustainable. You have control over the items that go into your meals when you cook at home, and you can ensure that your meals are nutritious and balanced. Cooking at home may also be a pleasant and gratifying pastime that can help you learn new cooking skills.

Mindful Eating is the discipline of paying attention to one's food and eating with purpose and mindfulness. By practicing mindful eating, you may learn to recognize your body's hunger and fullness signals and prevent overeating or eating when you're not hungry. Mindful eating may also help you experience the tastes and textures of the things you consume more thoroughly.

Get Creative: Eating a healthy diet does not have to be routine or boring. In truth, there are several ways to be creative with healthy eating and make it engaging and exciting. Experiment with new dishes, new fruits and vegetables, and new spices and tastes in your cooking. Making healthy eating more creative might assist to keep things interesting and minimize boredom or fatigue.

Find a Support System: Making healthy eating a habit may be difficult, and having a support system can be quite beneficial. Finding a friend or family member who shares your dedication to healthy eating, joining a healthy eating group or community, or obtaining help from a certified dietitian or other health experts may all help.

Chapter Two:

The Role of Exercise in Heart Health

The Value of Frequently Engaging in Physical Activity

In particular, when it comes to heart health, regular physical exercise is crucial for preserving good health and avoiding chronic illnesses. Blood is pumped by the heart throughout the body, providing cells and tissues with oxygen and nutrients. Regular exercise helps lower the risk of heart disease, stroke, and other cardiovascular problems by maintaining the heart's health and strength.

The following benefits of regular exercise are not the only ones that may improve heart health.

Reduces the Risk of Heart Disease: By lowering blood pressure, lowering blood cholesterol levels, and lowering the risk of diabetes, regular physical exercise may help to minimize the risk of heart disease. Additionally, it may aid in preventing artery-clogging plaque development that can result in heart attacks and strokes.

Strengthens the Heart Muscle: By strengthening the heart muscle, regular exercise may improve the heart's ability to pump blood more effectively throughout the body. Lessening the strain on the heart may lower the risk of heart disease and other cardiovascular diseases.

Regular exercise may aid to increase cardiovascular endurance, which makes it simpler for the heart to pump blood and oxygen to the body's tissues and organs. By doing so, you may feel less worn out and more healthy and happy overall.

Reduces Inflammation: Regular exercise may aid in reducing the body's overall inflammation, which can lead to the onset of chronic illnesses like heart disease. Regular exercise may enhance heart health and lower the risk of cardiovascular diseases by lowering inflammation.

Helps to regulate Weight: By burning calories and boosting metabolism, regular exercise may assist to regulate weight. Having too much weight may strain your heart, raising your risk of heart disease and other cardiovascular problems.

Reduces Stress: Stress and anxiety, which may contribute to the onset of heart disease and other chronic illnesses, can be lessened with regular physical exercise. Regular exercise may enhance heart health and general well-being by lowering stress.

Enhances Sleep: Regular exercise may assist to increase the quantity and quality of sleep, which can be beneficial for heart health. Improving sleep quality may be crucial for preserving heart health since it is linked to a lower risk of heart disease and other cardiovascular disorders.

Promotes General Well-Being: Regular exercise may assist to enhance general well-being, which helps support a healthy heart. Regular exercise may lower the risk of chronic illnesses like heart disease and other cardiovascular problems by enhancing general health.

Exercise Techniques for Cardiovascular Health

Exercise of many kinds, including aerobic activity, strength training, and high-intensity interval training (HIIT), may be beneficial to cardiovascular health. Every kind of exercise has certain advantages for heart health and general fitness.

Exercise that raises your heart rate and breathing rate is referred to as aerobic exercise or cardio exercise. When exercising aerobically, vast muscular groups are used repeatedly and rhythmically over an extended length of time. It is a crucial part of living a healthy lifestyle and has several advantages, such as enhancing cardiovascular health, boosting stamina, and lowering the risk of chronic illnesses.

Aerobic exercise types:

- Low-impact aerobics: An aerobic activity that is easy on the joints is low-impact aerobic exercise. To lessen the strain on the joints, this kind of exercise requires that one foot remains in constant touch with the ground. The low-impact aerobic workouts of walking, cycling, and swimming are examples.

- High-impact Aerobics: Compared to low-impact aerobic exercise, the high-impact aerobic activity includes greater hopping and bouncing. Exercises in this category include jogging, jumping jacks, and jumping rope.

- Step Aerobics: Step aerobics is a kind of aerobic exercise in which activities are carried out on a step or platform. Step aerobics is a vigorous exercise style that incorporates stepping, leaping, and kicking motions.

- Water Aerobics: In a swimming pool, water aerobics is a low-impact type of aerobic exercise. Moving while submerged in water creates resistance and lessens the pressure on the joints during this kind of workout. A great exercise for those with joint issues or injuries is water aerobics.

various forms of aerobic exercise

Walking: Walking is a simple, no-equipment-required, low-impact aerobic activity. Walking may be customized to suit various levels of fitness and can be done both inside and outdoors.

Running is a high-impact aerobic activity that may strengthen the heart and boost endurance. Running is an excellent method to lose weight and lower your chance of developing chronic conditions like diabetes, obesity, and heart disease.

Cycling is a low-impact aerobic activity that may be performed both indoors and outside. Cycling may strengthen stamina, boost cardiovascular health, and burn calories. Cycling may be done on a stationary cycle or a conventional bike and can be tailored to various fitness levels.

Swimming: Swimming is a low-impact, arthritic-friendly form of aerobic exercise. Swimming may strengthen stamina, boost cardiovascular health, and burn calories. You can swim in a lake, an ocean, or a pool.

Dancing: Dancing is a pleasurable and entertaining kind of aerobic exercise that may boost stamina, benefit cardiovascular health, and burn calories. Depending on your degree of fitness, you may dance by yourself or with a partner.

Jumping Rope: Jumping rope is a vigorous aerobic workout that increases stamina, strengthens the heart, and burns calories. Jump roping simply needs a jump rope and may be done both indoors and outside.

High-Intensity Interval Training (HIIT) is a kind of exercise that alternates brief bursts of vigorous activity with rest or low-intensity exercise. HIIT may enhance stamina, boost cardiovascular health, and burn calories.

Aerobic exercise has many advantages, including:

Increases blood flow and oxygen supply to the heart muscle, which improves heart health.

Reduces blood pressure and the risk of hypertension

Increases HDL (good) cholesterol while decreasing LDL (bad) cholesterol to improve cholesterol levels.

It aids in weight loss by burning calories and improving metabolism.

Reduces overall inflammation, which may lead to the development of heart disease and other chronic illnesses.

Resistance training, often known as strength training or weightlifting, is a kind of physical exercise in which weights or other types of resistance are used to increase muscular strength and endurance. Weight machines, free weights, resistance bands, and bodyweight exercises may all be used for resistance training. It is a crucial component of a well-rounded fitness regimen with several advantages, including increased muscle mass, bone density, and metabolic health.

Resistance exercise is also beneficial to cardiovascular health. Resistance exercise may assist to lower the risk of heart disease by decreasing numerous cardiovascular risk factors.

Resistance Training Categories:
Weight Machines: In many gyms, weight machines are a popular type of resistance training. These devices give a regulated exercise by using weight stacks or other types of resistance.

Free weights, such as dumbbells and barbells, are another common kind of resistance exercise. Weight machines need less stability than free weights, which might aid with balance and coordination.

Resistance bands are a convenient and inexpensive type of resistance training that may be utilized at home or on the road. Resistance bands are available in a variety of resistance levels, making them appropriate for people of various fitness levels.

Bodyweight Exercises: Push-ups, squats, and lunges are easy and efficient forms of resistance training that can be done anywhere. Bodyweight workouts do not need any equipment and may be adjusted to various fitness levels.

Here are some ways that resistance exercise might help your heart:

Reduces Blood Pressure: Hypertension is a key risk factor for heart disease. Resistance training has been found in studies to help lower blood pressure in both healthy and hypertensive persons. This is because resistance exercise induces blood vessels to widen, which improves blood flow and decreases the burden on the heart.

Improves Cholesterol Levels: High LDL ("bad") cholesterol levels and low HDL ("good") cholesterol levels are linked to an increased risk of heart disease. Resistance exercise has been demonstrated to lower LDL cholesterol while improving HDL cholesterol levels.

Inflammation is reduced: Chronic inflammation is a risk factor for heart disease. Resistance exercise has been found to lessen inflammation by lowering blood levels of inflammatory markers.

Insulin Sensitivity is Improved: Insulin resistance is a risk factor for type 2 diabetes, which is a risk factor for heart disease. Resistance training has been demonstrated to enhance insulin sensitivity, which may aid in the prevention of type 2 diabetes and heart disease.

Endothelial function is the lining of blood vessels, and endothelial dysfunction is a risk factor for heart disease. Resistance exercise has been demonstrated to enhance endothelial function, which increases blood flow and lowers the risk of heart disease.

Exercise Strategies to Incorporate Into Your Life

One of the most essential things you can do for your heart health is to exercise regularly. However, including exercise in your daily routine might be difficult, particularly if you have a hectic schedule or dislike conventional types of exercise.

The tactics listed here will not only help you include exercise in your daily routine, but they will also enhance your heart health.

Find an activity you love: Finding an exercise you enjoy is the key to adhering to a workout plan. Choose an activity that you like, whether it's walking, swimming, dancing, or playing sports. This will help you remain motivated and stick to a regular fitness schedule.

Set attainable objectives: Setting attainable goals might help you remain focused and motivated. Begin by creating simple, attainable objectives, such as walking for 30 minutes three times each week. Gradually increase the intensity and length of your exercises as you feel more comfortable with them.

Make exercise a priority: Making exercise a priority is essential for making it a regular part of your routine. Schedule your exercises around your schedule and regard them as appointments that must not be missed.

Include exercise in your everyday routine: Including exercise in your daily routine might help make it more doable. You could, for example, walk or cycle to work, use the stairs rather than the elevator or perform squats while brushing your teeth.

Participate in a fitness class or group: Participating in a fitness class or group may help with accountability and support. Having a group of people to exercise with, whether it's a yoga class, a running club, or a gym membership, may make it more pleasurable and help you remain motivated.

Utilize technology: There are several applications and fitness trackers available to assist you in tracking your progress and staying motivated. Using technology to measure your steps, calories burnt, or heart rate may help you remain on track and reach your fitness objectives.

Make it a family affair: Including physical activity in your family's routine will help everyone remain active and healthy. Finding things that everyone loves, whether it's going for a family stroll after dinner or playing a game of basketball together, may make fitness more pleasant and pleasurable.

Begin slowly and gradually increase your activity level: Starting slowly and gradually raising your activity level may help you prevent injury and burnout. Begin by exercising for

10-15 minutes each day and progressively increasing the time and intensity of your activities.

Variety is essential for remaining engaged and avoiding boredom. Include a combination of cardio and strength training in your regimen, and experiment with new activities and routines to keep things fresh.

Celebrate your victories: No matter how minor, celebrating your victories will help you remain inspired and devoted to your workout regimen. Take the time to notice and celebrate your accomplishments, whether it's completing a fitness milestone or just feeling more energetic and healthier.

Chapter Three:

The Role of Sleep in Heart Health

The Value of Sleep in Cardiovascular Health

Sleep is an important aspect of maintaining good heart health and is a vital part of leading a healthy lifestyle. Sleep not only makes us feel relaxed and rejuvenated, but it also plays an important part in the health of our cardiovascular system. A sufficient amount of sleep has been demonstrated to enhance cardiovascular function, decrease blood pressure, reduce inflammation, and minimize the risk of heart disease. Many individuals, however, struggle to get enough sleep, and sleep deprivation has become a serious public health problem.

The Relationship Between Sleep and Cardiovascular Health

According to research, obtaining adequate sleep is essential for maintaining healthy cardiovascular function. Sleep deprivation has been related to an increased risk of heart disease, stroke, and other cardiovascular problems. To maintain optimum heart health, the American Heart Association advises that individuals receive at least 7-8 hours of sleep every night.

Several critical activities occur in the body during sleep that aids in the maintenance of cardiovascular health. For example, during deep sleep, the body creates melatonin, a hormone that helps regulate blood pressure and heart rate. Furthermore, sleep is when the body repairs and regenerates cells, which is critical for maintaining healthy blood vessels and lowering inflammation.

The Importance of Getting Enough Sleep

Sleep Aids in Blood Pressure Regulation
Sleep is essential for managing blood pressure, which is a major risk factor for cardiovascular disease. During sleep, the body undergoes many physiological changes that aid in the reduction of blood pressure and the maintenance of normal levels. A drop in heart rate, a decrease in sympathetic nervous system activity, and an increase in parasympathetic nervous system activity are among the alterations.

When we sleep, our bodies enter a state of relaxation, enabling our heart rate to slow. A reduced heart rate lowers the quantity of blood pumped by the heart, resulting in a drop in blood pressure. During sleep, the body also creates more melatonin, a hormone that helps control blood pressure. Melatonin is a hormone generated by the pineal gland that promotes sleep and regulates the body's circadian cycles.

Sleep influences the synthesis of other hormones that control blood pressure, such as cortisol and adrenaline, in addition to melatonin. Cortisol is an adrenal gland hormone that helps control blood sugar levels and plays a function in the body's stress response. Adrenaline, often known as epinephrine, is a hormone generated by the adrenal glands that aid in physical preparation.

The body generates less cortisol and adrenaline during sleep, which helps to lower blood pressure. This is because these hormones induce blood vessels to contract, raising blood pressure. When the body is relaxed during sleep, the blood vessels may widen, lowering blood pressure.

Sleep also has an impact on the autonomic nervous system, which controls involuntary physiological activities including heart rate and blood pressure. The sympathetic nervous system and the parasympathetic nervous system are two branches of the autonomic nervous system. The sympathetic nervous system is in charge of the body's fight or flight reaction, which causes a rise in heart rate and blood pressure in response to stress. The parasympathetic nervous system, on the other hand, aids in relaxing by slowing the heart rate and blood pressure.

The sympathetic nervous system activity in the body diminishes during sleep, whereas the parasympathetic nervous system activity rises. This change in activity promotes relaxation and lowers blood pressure. Inadequate sleep, on the other hand, may upset this equilibrium and result in increased sympathetic nervous system activity, which can contribute to elevated blood pressure.

Furthermore, sleep influences the renin-angiotensin-aldosterone system, which is a hormonal mechanism that helps control blood pressure. Renin, a hormone released by the kidneys in reaction to low blood pressure or low blood volume, is involved in this mechanism. Renin aids in the conversion of the protein angiotensinogen into angiotensin I, which in turn is turned into angiotensin II, a hormone that constricts blood vessels and elevates blood pressure.

The renin-angiotensin-aldosterone system is repressed during sleep, which aids in the maintenance of normal blood pressure. Inadequate sleep or sleep disorders, such as sleep apnea, may wreak havoc on this system, leading to elevated blood pressure.

Sleep Aids in the Reduction of Inflammation
Sleep has an important role in controlling the body's inflammatory response. Although inflammation is a natural immunological response to injury or infection, it may also contribute to the development of many chronic disorders, including cardiovascular disease.

The body creates cytokines during sleep, which are substances that govern the immune system's response to inflammation. Sleep deprivation may impair cytokine synthesis, resulting in increased inflammation in the body.

People who habitually receive fewer than 6 hours of sleep every night have increased levels of inflammatory markers in their blood, such as C-reactive protein (CRP), interleukin-6 (IL-6), and tumor necrosis factor-alpha (TNF-alpha). These indicators are linked to an increased risk of cardiovascular disease and other chronic disorders.

Getting adequate sleep, on the other hand, may help decrease inflammation in the body. According to one research, increasing sleep duration by only one hour every night lowered CRP levels in the blood. Another research discovered that persons who slept for at least 7 hours each night had lower blood levels of inflammatory markers than those who slept for 6 hours or less.

Sleep also helps to regulate the body's stress response, which may lead to inflammation. Chronic stress may raise cortisol levels, a hormone that causes inflammation. Getting adequate sleep may aid in the regulation of cortisol levels and the reduction of inflammation in the body.

Sleep may also assist manage the gut flora, which is important for immune function and inflammation. Chronic inflammation and an increased risk of chronic illnesses, including heart disease, have been related to gut microbiota disruption. Sleep deprivation may upset the gut microbiome's equilibrium, resulting in increased inflammation in the body.

Sleep Aids in Blood Sugar Control
Sleep is essential for controlling blood sugar levels in the body. Insulin is a hormone that controls blood sugar levels by promoting glucose absorption from the circulation into the cells of the body, where it may be utilized for energy or stored as glycogen. Sleep deprivation may cause insulin resistance and impair insulin synthesis, increasing the risk of developing type 2 diabetes.

The body's metabolic activities slow down during sleep, allowing for tissue healing and regeneration. This involves restoring insulin sensitivity and controlling glucose metabolism.

Sleep deprivation may alter these mechanisms, resulting in lower insulin sensitivity and higher blood sugar levels.

People who habitually receive fewer than 6 hours of sleep each night have greater levels of blood sugar and insulin resistance than those who get 7-8 hours of sleep per night, according to studies. According to one research, healthy young individuals who were sleep deprived for only one night had an increase in insulin resistance and blood sugar levels the following day.

Sleep also helps to regulate the body's synthesis of blood sugar-regulating chemicals including cortisol and growth hormone. Cortisol is a stress hormone that can raise blood sugar levels. Growth hormone, on the other hand, aids in the regulation of glucose metabolism and the absorption of glucose by the body's cells. These hormone disruptions may lead to elevated blood sugar levels and an increased risk of developing type 2 diabetes.

Furthermore, sleep may influence food intake and appetite management, both of which affect blood sugar levels. Sleep deprivation may impair the body's synthesis of appetite-regulating hormones such as leptin and ghrelin. Leptin is a hormone that indicates satiety, while ghrelin is a hunger hormone. Disruption of these hormones may result in increased food intake and cravings for high-sugar and high-carbohydrate meals, both of which can contribute to elevated blood sugar levels.

Sleep, in addition to controlling blood sugar levels, is important for general metabolic health. Obesity, metabolic syndrome, and cardiovascular disease have all been related to chronic sleep deprivation, all of which are risk factors for type 2 diabetes.

Sleep Aids in Weight Maintenance
Sleep is essential for keeping a healthy weight. An increasing amount of evidence demonstrates that enough sleep is critical for obtaining and maintaining a healthy weight.

This is because sleep is essential for regulating the body's metabolism, hunger, and energy expenditure.

Sleep aids in the maintenance of a healthy weight by modulating the hormones that govern appetite and fullness. Leptin is a hormone generated by fat cells that alerts the brain when the body's energy reserves are depleted. Ghrelin is a hormone generated by the stomach that alerts the brain to hunger. Sleep deprivation may interfere with the synthesis of these hormones, causing an increase in hunger and food consumption. According to studies, persons who sleep fewer than 6 hours per night had greater ghrelin levels and lower leptin levels than those who sleep 7-9 hours per night.

Sleep also helps to maintain a healthy weight by regulating the body's metabolism. The body's metabolic rate slows down during sleep, allowing it to preserve energy and promote tissue repair and development. Chronic sleep deprivation may cause a drop in metabolism, making it more difficult for the body to burn calories and maintain a healthy weight.

Furthermore, sleep loss may cause an increase in the body's synthesis of cortisol, a stress hormone. High cortisol levels may contribute to increased fat accumulation in the body, especially in the abdomen. This may lead to a rise in body weight and an increased risk of obesity-related health issues including type 2 diabetes and cardiovascular disease.

In addition, a lack of sleep may cause exhaustion and a loss of willingness to participate in physical exercise. Exercise is essential for keeping a healthy weight, and persistent sleep deprivation may make it more difficult to participate in regular physical exercise. This may lead to weight gain and a reduced capacity to maintain a healthy weight.

Sleep Disorders and Heart Health

A sleep disturbance is a medical illness that interferes with the quality, timing, and duration of sleep, resulting in difficulty falling asleep, remaining asleep, or waking up too early. Medical illnesses, drugs, environmental variables, and lifestyle behaviors may all contribute to sleep disturbances. Insomnia, obstructive sleep apnea, restless leg syndrome, and narcolepsy are all common sleep disorders. These illnesses may have serious consequences for one's general health and well-being, including mental health, cardiovascular health, and cognitive function. Depending on the underlying cause of the condition, treatment for sleep disturbances may include lifestyle modifications, medication, or counseling.

The Effects of Sleep Disorders on Heart Health

Obstructive Sleep Apnea (OSA) is a sleep condition in which the airway contracts regularly during sleep, causing breathing to stop and resume periodically during the night. OSA is a widespread problem that affects around 22 million Americans and is linked to many negative health implications, including an increased risk of heart disease.

When the airway gets closed during an episode of OSA, the brain is deprived of oxygen, leading the body to respond by releasing stress hormones like adrenaline. This stress reaction may cause a variety of physiological changes that can have a long-term harmful influence on the heart and cardiovascular system.

OSA may have a substantial influence on heart health by contributing to the development of excessive blood pressure, or hypertension. According to research, those with OSA are up to three times more likely to develop hypertension than those who do not have the disorder. Because repeated bouts of breathing stoppage during sleep may cause blood oxygen levels to plummet, stress hormones are released, which can constrict blood vessels and elevate blood pressure.

This high blood pressure may damage the artery walls over time, increasing the risk of major cardiovascular events such as heart attack, stroke, and heart failure. Research has revealed that those with untreated OSA are more likely to develop cardiovascular disease and have a cardiovascular event than those who do not have the illness.

OSA may cause changes in the structure and function of the heart, in addition to contributing to the development of hypertension. People with OSA are more likely to develop an enlarged heart, known as left ventricular hypertrophy, which is a typical prelude to heart failure, according to research. OSA may also affect changes in the way the heart beats and decrease the heart's capacity to adequately pump blood.

Other ways that OSA may harm heart health include causing arrhythmias, or abnormal heartbeats, and impairing the body's ability to manage blood sugar levels. Furthermore, OSA has been linked to an increased chance of obesity, which is another key risk factor for heart disease.

Treatment
Fortunately, a variety of effective therapies for OSA are available, which may help improve

both sleep quality and heart health. Constant Positive Airway Pressure (CPAP) therapy is one of the most used treatments for OSA. It entails sleeping with a mask over the nose or mouth that provides a constant stream of air to keep the airway open.

Other therapies for OSA may include weight loss, abstaining from alcohol and sedatives, and sleeping on one's side, as well as surgical procedures such as uvulopalatopharyngoplasty (UPPP) or the installation of a dental device to keep the airway open.

Aside from these therapies, other lifestyle adjustments, such as eating a nutritious diet, exercising regularly, and managing stress, may help improve both sleep quality and heart health. Individuals may minimize their chance of developing heart disease and other significant health concerns related to OSA by treating it and adopting other beneficial adjustments.

Insomnia is a prevalent sleep problem that affects millions of individuals throughout the globe. It is distinguished by difficulties going asleep, remaining asleep, or waking up too early and being unable to return to sleep. Insomnia may be acute (for a few days or weeks) or persistent (for months or years). While a single sleepless night may not be harmful, persistent insomnia may have substantial consequences for both physical and mental health, including an increased chance of developing heart disease.

Insomnia may have many negative effects on heart health:

Chronic insomnia may result in a continuous rise in blood pressure, which can damage the arteries and raise the risk of heart disease.

Reduced Heart Rate Variability (HRV): HRV refers to the fluctuation in time between consecutive heartbeats. It is a crucial indication of cardiovascular health, and low HRV has been related to an increased risk of cardiovascular disease. It has been shown that insomnia reduces HRV, which may lead to an increased risk of heart disease.

Insomnia has been associated with an increase in inflammatory markers in the body. Inflammation is a recognized risk factor for heart disease since it may cause artery damage and increase the likelihood of plaque accumulation.

Obesity Risk: Insomnia has been related to an increased risk of obesity. Obesity, which may lead to high blood pressure, high cholesterol, and diabetes, is a recognized risk factor for heart disease.

Insomnia has been related to an increased chance of acquiring type 2 diabetes, which is a recognized risk factor for heart disease.

Heart Attack and Stroke Risk elevated: Chronic sleeplessness has been related to an elevated risk of heart attack and stroke. This is assumed to be owing to the effect of insomnia on blood pressure, inflammation, and other risk factors for cardiovascular disease.

Treatment
Cognitive Behavioral Therapy (CBT): CBT is a sort of talk therapy that may help with insomnia. It entails recognizing and altering unfavorable thinking patterns and actions that may be related to sleep issues.

Sleep Hygiene: Good sleep practices that may assist enhance the quality and amount of sleep are referred to as sleep hygiene. Setting a regular sleep routine, avoiding coffee and alcohol before bed, and having a pleasant sleep environment are all part of this.

drugs: Benzodiazepines, non-benzodiazepine sedatives, and melatonin agonists are among the drugs that may be used to treat insomnia. These drugs should only be taken under the supervision of a healthcare practitioner since they may cause negative effects and interact with other medications.

Alternative treatments: Acupuncture, yoga, and meditation are three alternative treatments that may be useful in treating insomnia. These treatments may aid in the promotion of relaxation and the improvement of sleep quality.

RLS (Restless Leg Syndrome):
RLS is a neurological disorder that causes an insatiable need to move one's legs. This impulse is generally accompanied by an unpleasant sensation, such as crawling, itching, or burning. These feelings may range from moderate to severe, and they differ from person to person.

RLS may affect anybody, although women and adults over the age of 40 are more likely to suffer from it. RLS has no established etiology, however it is thought to be caused by a malfunction in the brain's dopamine system, which governs movement and feelings in the body.

RLS symptoms usually appear at night and may drastically impair sleep habits. This might cause exhaustion, sleepiness, and irritation throughout the day, which can have a detrimental influence on everyday activities.

The Relationship Between Restless Leg Syndrome and Cardiovascular Health

Recent studies have revealed a link between RLS and an increased risk of heart disease. While the specific nature of the link is unknown, multiple studies have suggested that patients with RLS are more likely to acquire cardiovascular disease.

According to one research published in the journal Sleep Medicine, those with RLS had a 1.5-fold greater risk of getting heart disease compared to those who do not have the illness. Another research published in the journal Circulation discovered that persons with RLS were more likely to develop hypertension, which is a key risk factor for heart disease.

The precise mechanism behind this link is yet unknown. However, it is thought that RLS-induced sleep disturbance may play a role. Sleep is critical for cardiovascular health, and changes in sleep patterns may result in increased inflammation, oxidative stress, and other variables that can contribute to the development of heart disease.

Several RLS-related conditions might have a harmful influence on heart health. These are some examples:

RLS may drastically disturb sleep patterns, resulting in exhaustion, sleepiness, and irritability throughout the day. Chronic sleep disturbance has been associated with an increased risk of cardiovascular illness, such as hypertension, stroke, and heart attack.

Hypertension
RLS and hypertension have been linked in many studies. Hypertension is a key risk factor for heart disease and stroke, and those with RLS may be more likely to acquire it.

Syndrome Metabolique
excessive blood pressure, excessive blood sugar, excess body fat, and abnormal cholesterol levels are all symptoms of metabolic syndrome. People with RLS may be more likely to develop

metabolic syndrome, which increases the risk of heart disease considerably.

Treatment
Medications
Several drugs are available to help relieve RLS symptoms. These include dopamine agonists, which assist control dopamine levels in the brain, and iron supplements, which may help those with iron deficiency reduce symptoms.

Changes in Lifestyle
Modifications to one's daily routine, behavior, and habits that might contribute to a healthy lifestyle are referred to as lifestyle adjustments. Adopting good dietary habits, regular exercise, stress management, and getting adequate sleep are examples of these improvements. Lifestyle changes have a substantial influence on general health and are often advised as part of the treatment plan for a variety of medical issues, including heart disease.

Methods for Improving Your Sleeping Habits

Maintain a consistent sleep routine.

Sticking to a regular sleep schedule is one of the most important things you can do to enhance your sleep patterns. Even on weekends, going to bed and getting up at the same time every day helps to regulate your body's internal clock and promotes greater sleep quality. Aim for seven to eight hours of sleep every night, and avoid staying up late or sleeping in on weekends.

Make a soothing nighttime ritual.

Creating a peaceful bedtime ritual may assist in signaling to your body that it is time to wind down and prepare for sleep. Activities like taking a warm bath, reading a book, or practicing relaxation methods such as deep breathing or meditation fall under this category. Avoid stimulating activities such as watching television or using your phone since the blue light generated by electronic gadgets might disrupt your body's normal sleep-wake cycle.

Make your sleeping surroundings as comfy as possible.

The quality of your sleeping environment might have a big influence on your sleep quality. Assemble a cool, quiet, and comfy bedroom, complete with a sturdy mattress and pillows. You may also consider investing in blackout curtains or an eye mask to filter out any light that might interfere with your sleep.

Limit your midday naps.
While taking a nap during the day might be appealing, particularly if you're exhausted, it can interfere with your ability to sleep at night. If you must nap, keep it to 20-30 minutes and try to schedule it in the early afternoon.

Caffeine and alcohol should be avoided.
Caffeine and alcohol may disrupt your sleep, so it's better to avoid them or restrict your use. Caffeine should be avoided in the afternoon and evening since it may persist in your system for up to 12 hours. Although alcohol may make you feel tired at first, it may impair your sleep later in the night.

Exercise regularly.

Regular exercise, when done at the proper time, may assist promote improved sleep quality. Exercise at least three hours before night because it produces endorphins, which might make it harder to fall asleep quickly. Exercise regularly may help enhance cardiovascular health and lower the risk of heart disease.

Control your stress levels.

Stress may impair your ability to fall and remain asleep, so it's important to discover techniques to regulate your stress levels. Deep breathing, meditation, yoga, and therapy are examples of such practices. It's also beneficial to build a calm nighttime ritual and a comfy sleeping environment.

Large meals should be avoided before going to bed.

A heavy meal before night might make it difficult to fall asleep and raise your risk of heartburn or acid reflux. If you must eat within two to three hours of going to bed, limit yourself to tiny, light snacks.

Blue light exposure should be limited.
As previously stated, blue light generated by electronic gadgets such as phones and tablets might disrupt your sleep. Limit your nighttime blue light exposure by shutting off electronic devices or utilizing blue light filters on your gadgets.

Seek medical help.
If you've tried these measures and are still having trouble sleeping, it's time to consult a doctor. Your doctor may be able to uncover any underlying medical disorders that are interfering with your sleep or offer medications to help you sleep better.

Chapter Four:

The Role of Stress Management in Heart Health

Stress's Influence on Cardiovascular Health

Stress is a natural aspect of life and is the body's reaction to a difficult or dangerous circumstance. Stress causes the body to release chemicals such as adrenaline and cortisol, which may cause physical and psychological changes. While short-term stress might be beneficial in certain instances, persistent stress can be harmful to one's cardiovascular health.

Stress may have a variety of effects on the cardiovascular system. It may, for example, trigger the production of stress hormones, which causes an increase in heart rate, blood pressure, and blood sugar levels. These modifications may strain the heart and raise the risk of heart disease.

Chronic stress may also have an impact on the immune system, causing inflammation that can damage blood vessels and contribute to the development of atherosclerosis. Atherosclerosis is a disorder in which plaque accumulates in the arteries, narrowing them and making them less flexible, increasing the risk of heart attacks and strokes.

Stress may also lead to harmful habits like smoking, overeating, and not getting enough exercise, all of which can lead to poor cardiovascular health.

Chronic stress, according to research, puts people at a greater risk of getting cardiovascular disease. According to research published in the Journal of the American College of Cardiology, those who reported high levels of stress at work had a 48% higher chance of developing atrial fibrillation, a form of irregular heartbeat that may raise the risk of stroke.

Furthermore, research published in the European Heart Journal found that those who reported high levels of stress had a 27% higher risk of heart disease and a 48% higher chance of dying from heart disease.

Techniques for Stress Management and Relaxation

For general cardiovascular health, it is critical to control stress and encourage relaxation.
These approaches will assist you with stress management and relaxation:

Meditation for Mindfulness

Mindfulness meditation is a practice that includes paying attention to the present moment and being aware of thoughts, emotions, and body sensations without judgment. This method has been demonstrated to reduce stress and increase general well-being. According to one research, mindfulness meditation may considerably reduce blood pressure in persons who have hypertension. A few minutes of mindfulness meditation incorporated into your daily routine may have a major influence on your overall stress levels.

Yoga

Yoga is a kind of exercise that incorporates physical postures, breathing methods, and meditation to achieve relaxation and stress reduction. Yoga has been demonstrated in studies to considerably reduce stress hormones like cortisol, lower blood pressure, and enhance overall cardiovascular health. Even a few minutes of yoga practice every day may have a major impact on stress reduction and relaxation.

Exercises in Deep Breathing

Deep breathing exercises are a simple and efficient method of reducing stress and promoting relaxation. The body's natural relaxation response is induced by concentrating on calm, deep breathing, resulting in a drop in heart rate and blood pressure. This approach may be used at any time and from any location, making it a practical alternative for regulating stress levels throughout the day.

Muscle Relaxation in Stages

Progressive muscle relaxation is a stress-reduction method that includes tensing and relaxing certain muscle groups. Individuals may become more aware of their physical and mental states by concentrating on the feelings of tension and relaxation in their bodies, resulting in a reduction in overall stress levels. This strategy has been found in studies to be beneficial in lowering anxiety and inducing relaxation.

Tai Chi

Tai Chi is a kind of exercise that combines mild physical motions, breathing methods, and meditation to achieve relaxation and stress reduction. Tai chi practice has been demonstrated in studies to considerably decrease stress, lower blood pressure, and enhance general cardiovascular health. Incorporating tai chi into your daily routine may have a big influence on stress management and relaxation.

Music Treatment

Music therapy is the practice of listening to music to aid relaxation and stress reduction. Listening to relaxing music has been found in studies to considerably decrease stress chemicals such as cortisol and blood pressure. Including music in your daily routine may be a fun and effective approach to reducing stress and promoting relaxation.

Acupuncture

Acupuncture is a treatment that includes putting tiny needles into certain body locations to induce relaxation and stress reduction. Acupuncture has been demonstrated in studies to be beneficial in decreasing stress and anxiety, as well as lowering blood pressure. Acupuncture may be an excellent approach to induce relaxation and lower stress levels if you include it in your stress management program.

Mind-Body Techniques for Cardiovascular Health

The mind-body link is widely documented, and research has shown that using mind-body activities may assist increase general health and wellness, including cardiovascular health. These activities attempt to promote relaxation, mental well-being, and stress reduction, all of which may benefit heart health. Here are a few mind-body techniques that may help with heart health:

Meditation entails concentrating on the present moment and obtaining a profound level of calm. This may be accomplished through a variety of approaches, including mindfulness meditation, transcendental meditation, and loving-kindness meditation. Regular meditation has been demonstrated in studies to help lower blood pressure, enhance heart rate variability, and lower the risk of heart disease.

Deep breathing techniques, such as diaphragmatic breathing and alternate nostril breathing, may aid in stress reduction and relaxation. These procedures may be used at any time and in any location, making them a simple and convenient approach to enhancing heart health.

Guided imagery is the use of visualization to aid relaxation and stress reduction. This may be accomplished by using guided meditations or envisioning soothing sights or circumstances. Guided imagery has been demonstrated in studies to help decrease stress, lower blood pressure, and increase heart rate variability.

Progressive muscle relaxation is tensing and then releasing various muscle groups in the body to encourage relaxation and stress reduction. This approach is beneficial in lowering stress and increasing sleep quality, both of which may benefit heart health.

Biofeedback is the use of technology to monitor physiological processes such as heart rate, blood pressure, and muscular tension to promote relaxation and reduce stress. This approach has been demonstrated to help lower blood pressure and improve heart rate variability.

Chapter Five:

Types of Heart Disease

Coronary Artery Disease

Coronary artery disease (CAD) is a frequent disorder where the arteries that feed blood to the heart become constricted or clogged. This may lead to a variety of consequences, including chest discomfort, heart attacks, and even heart failure. CAD is one of the top causes of mortality globally, yet it can typically be avoided or treated via a mix of lifestyle modifications, medication, and surgical treatments.

Heart Failure

Heart failure is a disorder that develops when the heart muscle is weakened or injured, making it harder for the heart to pump blood properly. This may lead to several symptoms, including shortness of breath, exhaustion, swelling in the legs and feet, and trouble exercising. While heart failure may be a severe illness, there are a variety of therapies and lifestyle adjustments that can help control the symptoms and improve the overall quality of life.

Causes of Heart Failure

Heart failure may be caused by a variety of reasons, including:

- Coronary artery disease
- High blood pressure
- Cardiomyopathy
- Heart valve disease
- Congenital heart defects
- Other factors: Other conditions that might lead to heart failure include diabetes, obesity, smoking, and alcohol misuse.

Symptoms of Heart Failure

The symptoms of heart failure may vary depending on the severity of the ailment, but frequent symptoms include:

- Shortness of breath: This is generally the first sign of heart failure and may occur during physical activity or while laying down.

- exhaustion: Many persons with heart failure report exhaustion, even when they have not pushed themselves.

- Swelling: Swelling in the legs, ankles, or feet is prevalent in persons with heart failure.

- Rapid or irregular heartbeat: This might be an indication that the heart is straining to pump blood adequately.

- Chest discomfort: Chest pain may arise if the heart is not getting enough oxygen.

Arrhythmias

Arrhythmias, commonly known as irregular heartbeats or heart rhythm disorders, refer to any variation from the normal rhythm of the heart. In a healthy heart, electrical impulses are transmitted by the sinoatrial (SA) node, the heart's natural pacemaker, which causes the contraction of the heart muscles and results in a heartbeat. However, in people with arrhythmias, this electrical activity is erratic, leading to either too rapid or too slow a pulse. Arrhythmias may vary from innocuous to life-threatening and can develop at any age.

There are numerous forms of arrhythmias, which are categorized depending on the location of the irregular heartbeat inside the heart, such as atrial fibrillation (AFib), supraventricular tachycardia (SVT), ventricular fibrillation (VFib), ventricular tachycardia (VTach).

AFib is the most prevalent kind of arrhythmia, impacting millions of individuals globally. It happens when the atria, the upper chambers of the heart, pulse unevenly, resulting in an irregular heartbeat. This syndrome may lead to blood clots, stroke, and heart failure.

SVT, on the other hand, refers to fast heartbeats that originate in the upper chambers of the heart. This condition may come rapidly and may induce dizziness, chest discomfort, and fainting.

VFib and VTach are potentially life-threatening arrhythmias that affect the ventricles, the bottom chambers of the heart. VFib is a chaotic and disorganized heartbeat that may lead to abrupt cardiac arrest, whereas VTach is a fast heartbeat that can result in fainting or cardiac arrest.

Arrhythmias may arise owing to many causes, including underlying cardiac disease, electrolyte imbalances, stress, excessive blood pressure, and drug or alcohol addiction. Certain drugs, such as beta-blockers and calcium channel blockers, may potentially lead to arrhythmias.

Symptoms of arrhythmias vary based on the nature and severity of the illness. Some persons with arrhythmias may not have any symptoms, while others may feel palpitations, chest discomfort, dizziness, fainting, or shortness of breath.

Valvular Heart Disease (VHD)

Valvular heart disease (VHD) refers to any ailment that affects the heart's valves, which govern the flow of blood through the chambers of the heart. When the valves are damaged or sick, they can't open or shut correctly, resulting in blood flow issues and other consequences. In this post, we will cover the causes, symptoms, diagnosis, and treatment options for valvular heart disease.

Causes of Valvular Heart Disease:

Valvular heart disease may be caused by many reasons, including congenital heart abnormalities, infections, or age-related wear and tear on the valves. Some frequent causes of valvular heart disease include:

- Congenital heart defects
- Age-related wear and tear: As individuals age, the heart valves may become thicker, stiff, or calcified, leading to valvular heart disease.
- Rheumatic fever: Rheumatic fever is a consequence of untreated strep throat that may cause inflammation and scarring of the heart valves.
- Endocarditis: Endocarditis is an infection of the inner lining of the heart that may damage the heart valves.

- Other problems: Valvular heart disease may also be caused by factors such as excessive blood pressure, coronary artery disease, and connective tissue abnormalities.

Symptoms of Valvular Heart Disease:

The symptoms of valvular heart disease might vary depending on the severity of the problem and which valves are impacted. Some typical signs of valvular heart disease include:

- Shortness of breath: This may occur during physical activity or even during rest.

- Fatigue: This might occur owing to reduced blood flow and oxygen to the body.

- Chest pain: This might develop owing to the reduced blood supply to the heart.

- Dizziness or fainting: This might occur owing to the reduced blood supply to the brain.

- Swelling of the legs, ankles, or feet: This may develop owing to fluid accumulation in the body.

Congenital Heart Disease (CHD)

Congenital heart disease (CHD) is a form of heart disease that arises when a newborn is born with a defective heart structure or function. It is the most prevalent kind of birth defect, affecting around 1% of all live births. Congenital heart disease may vary from basic problems that may not need treatment to severe diseases that require surgery or other treatments.

Causes of Congenital Heart Disease:

Congenital cardiac disease may be caused by several reasons, including genetic, environmental, and developmental factors. Some risk factors for the congenital cardiac disease include:

- Family history of congenital heart disease
- Maternal sickness during pregnancy
- Exposure to certain medicines or poisons during pregnancy
- Chromosomal abnormalities such as Down syndrome
- Advanced maternal age

Types of Congenital Heart Disease:

There are several forms of congenital heart disease, which may be categorized depending on the abnormality and the particular cardiac parts involved. Some of the most prevalent kinds of the congenital cardiac disease include:

Atrial septal defect (ASD): A hole in the wall between the two upper chambers of the heart. Ventricular septal defect (VSD): A hole in the wall between the two lower chambers of the heart.

Tetralogy of Fallot: A collection of four abnormalities that damage the heart's structure and function.

Transposition of the great arteries: A condition in which the two main arteries exiting the heart are swapped.

Coarctation of the aorta: A narrowing of the aorta, the major artery that transports blood from the heart to the body.

Symptoms of Congenital Heart Disease:

The symptoms of congenital cardiac disease might vary depending on the degree and kind of abnormality. Some newborns may have no symptoms at all, while others may develop severe problems quickly after delivery.

Some common signs of congenital heart disease include:

- Rapid breathing
- Poor feeding
- Cyanosis (a bluish tinge to the skin, lips, or fingernails)
- Fatigue or weakness during physical activity
- Chest pain
- Dizziness or fainting

Cardiomyopathy

Cardiomyopathy is a disease that damages the heart muscles. It makes it difficult for the heart to pump blood to the rest of the body, and it may progress to heart failure. Cardiomyopathy may be caused by numerous reasons, including hereditary factors, infections, and lifestyle decisions.

There are various forms of cardiomyopathy, including dilated cardiomyopathy, hypertrophic cardiomyopathy, and restrictive cardiomyopathy. Each variety has its origins, symptoms, and treatment choices.

Dilated Cardiomyopathy

Dilated cardiomyopathy is the most frequent kind of cardiomyopathy. It happens when the left ventricle of the heart gets enlarged and weaker, making it harder for the heart to pump blood adequately. This may lead to cardiac failure, arrhythmias, and other problems.

Various reasons may lead to the development of dilated cardiomyopathy, including genetics, infections, alcohol consumption, and drug usage. Other risk factors include hypertension, diabetes, and thyroid disorders.

Symptoms of dilated cardiomyopathy might include shortness of breath, weariness, swelling in the legs, ankles, or feet, and irregular heartbeat. In certain circumstances, individuals may not feel any symptoms until the illness has advanced.

Hypertrophic Cardiomyopathy

Hypertrophic cardiomyopathy is a hereditary disorder that causes the heart muscles to grow thicker, making it harder for the heart to pump blood adequately. It is one of the most prevalent causes of sudden cardiac death in young individuals.

Hypertrophic cardiomyopathy is caused by abnormalities in genes that affect the development and shape of the heart muscles. It may be inherited from one or both parents.

Symptoms of hypertrophic cardiomyopathy might include shortness of breath, chest discomfort, disorientation, and fainting. In certain circumstances, individuals may not feel any symptoms.

Restrictive Cardiomyopathy

Restrictive cardiomyopathy occurs when the heart muscles become stiff and tight, making it harder for the heart to pump blood adequately. It is the rarest kind of cardiomyopathy.

Restrictive cardiomyopathy may be caused by numerous reasons, including amyloidosis, sarcoidosis, and hemochromatosis. These disorders cause the cardiac muscles to get invaded with aberrant substances, making them stiff and unyielding.

Symptoms of restrictive cardiomyopathy might include shortness of breath, tiredness, and swelling in the legs, ankles, or feet. In certain circumstances, individuals may not feel any symptoms.

Aortic aneurysm

An aortic aneurysm is a significant medical disorder that may have life-threatening effects if left untreated. It happens when there is a bulge or weakness in the wall of the aorta, the biggest artery in the body, that may lead to a rupture or dissection. Aortic aneurysms may form anywhere along the aorta but are most typically encountered in the abdominal or thoracic regions. In this post, we will cover the causes, symptoms, diagnosis, and treatment options for aortic aneurysms.

Causes of Aortic Aneurysm:
The specific causes of aortic aneurysms are not yet completely known, however, some risk factors have been found. These include:

- Age: The chance of having an aortic aneurysm rises with age, particularly beyond the age of 60.

- Smoking: Cigarette smoking is a substantial risk factor for aortic aneurysms, since it may cause damage to the walls of the aorta.

- High blood pressure: Uncontrolled high blood pressure may lead to the weakening of the aorta walls, increasing the risk of an aneurysm.

- Atherosclerosis: An accumulation of plaque in the arteries may potentially compromise the aortic walls, leading to an aneurysm.

- Family history: A family history of aortic aneurysms might raise the chance of acquiring one.

Symptoms of Aortic Aneurysm:

In many situations, aortic aneurysms do not produce any symptoms and are only detected inadvertently during imaging investigations for other illnesses. However, if symptoms do emerge, they might include:

- Chest or back pain: This might be a symptom of a dissection or rupture of the aneurysm.

- Abdominal pain: This is a frequent sign of an abdominal aortic aneurysm.

- Difficulty breathing: This might occur if the aneurysm is pushing on the lungs or airways.

- Hoarseness: This might develop if the aneurysm is pushing on the nerves that regulate the vocal cords.

- Swelling: This may develop in the legs or belly if the aneurysm is big enough to restrict blood flow.

Chapter Six:

Cardiovascular Disease Risk Factors

Any condition or action that raises the likelihood of acquiring cardiovascular disease is referred to as a risk factor for heart disease. Several risk factors have a role in its development. Some of these risk factors are within your control, while others are not. Understanding these risk factors may assist people in taking efforts to lower their risk and preserve their heart health. In this post, we will look at the different risk factors for heart disease and how they affect cardiovascular health.

Risk Factors that can be modified or controlled

High Blood Pressure: A frequent risk factor for heart disease is high blood pressure. Blood pressure is the force of blood on the walls of the arteries, and it may damage the arteries and raise the risk of developing heart disease if it is regularly high. Controlling blood pressure with medication, lifestyle modifications, and frequent monitoring may lower the chance of getting heart disease greatly.

High Cholesterol: High cholesterol levels in the blood may cause plaque to build in the arteries, increasing the risk of heart disease. Controlling cholesterol levels with medication, food, and lifestyle modifications may lower the chance of developing heart disease.

Diabetes is a disease that impairs the body's capacity to manage blood sugar levels. Diabetes increases the chance of developing heart disease because high blood sugar may damage blood arteries and neurons. Blood sugar control with medication, food, and lifestyle modifications may help minimize the chance of developing heart disease.

Tobacco use is a major risk factor for heart disease because it destroys blood vessels, raises blood pressure, and limits oxygen supply to the heart. Quitting smoking may cut the chance of getting heart disease considerably.

Obesity: Due to the pressure on the heart and blood arteries, being overweight or obese might raise the chance of getting heart disease. Losing weight via diet and exercise may lower the chance of having heart disease dramatically.

Sedentism: A sedentary lifestyle raises the chance of acquiring heart disease. Exercise regularly may help lower the chance of developing heart disease and improve overall cardiovascular health.

Unhealthy eating habits
A diet heavy in saturated fats, trans fats, salt, and added sweets may raise the risk of heart disease.

Fruits, vegetables, whole grains, lean meats, and healthy fats found in nuts, seeds, and fish are all part of a heart-healthy diet. Limiting your consumption of processed meals, sugary beverages, and foods rich in saturated and trans fats will help lower your risk of developing heart disease.

Non-modifiable risk factor or Risk factors that cannot be altered

Non-modifiable risk factors for heart disease are those that a person cannot modify or control. These risk factors are often linked to genetic and environmental variables over which we have no control. While non-modifiable risk factors cannot be modified, people may take actions to minimize their overall risk of heart disease by being aware of them. Some of the most frequent non-modifiable risk factors for heart disease are as follows:

Age: The risk of heart disease rises with age. This is because our arteries grow less flexible and narrower with time, making it more difficult for blood to flow through them. Heart disease is more common in males over the age of 45 and in women over the age of 55.

Gender: Men are more likely than premenopausal women to have heart disease. However, following menopause, women's risk of heart disease rises to that of males.

A close family member who has had heart disease increases the likelihood of having it. This is because hereditary factors might contribute to the development of heart disease.

Ethnicity: Certain ethnic groups, such as African Americans, Mexican Americans, American Indians, and certain Asian Americans, are at a greater risk of having heart disease.

Previous heart attack or stroke: People who have had a previous heart attack or stroke are more likely to have another one.

Congenital heart problems: Some people are born with structural heart abnormalities that raise their chance of developing heart disease later in life.

Individuals may still take action to minimize their overall risk of heart disease even if non-modifiable risk factors cannot be addressed. This involves concentrating on controllable risk factors including eating a nutritious diet and exercising regularly, managing stress, and quitting smoking. Working with a healthcare professional to build a tailored strategy for lowering the risk of heart disease based on individual risk factors and overall health status is critical. Regular check-ups and screenings may also aid in the detection of early indicators of heart disease, allowing for early intervention and treatment.

Chapter Seven:

Diagnosis and Treatment of Heart Disease

Heart Disease Diagnostic Tests

Early identification is critical for successful management and therapy. Diagnostic tests for heart disease assist healthcare practitioners determine the kind and severity of the ailment, allowing them to build a specific treatment strategy. A detailed medical history and physical examination are the initial steps in identifying cardiac disease. Your symptoms, medical history, and family history of heart disease will be discussed with the doctor. Listening to your heart and lungs, as well as monitoring your blood pressure and pulse, will be part of the physical exam.

Your doctor may offer several tests to assist identify heart disease in addition to a medical history and physical examination. Among these tests are:

Electrocardiogram.
A non-invasive test that monitors the electrical activity of the heart is known as an electrocardiogram. Electrodes are attached to the chest, arms, and legs to record the electrical impulses of the heart. Arrhythmias, heart attacks, heart enlargement, and irregular cardiac rhythms may all be detected with an ECG.

The echocardiogram (Echo)
An echocardiogram is a non-invasive test that creates pictures of the heart using sound waves. The examination measures the size and shape of the heart, as well as its pumping performance and blood flow. An echocardiogram may reveal problems with the heart valves, heart walls, and blood arteries.

Stress Test Through Exercise

An exercise stress test assesses the function of the heart during physical exertion. Walking on a treadmill or riding a stationary bike while attached to ECG equipment is part of the exam. The test assesses the heart's reaction to stress, giving data on blood flow and diagnosing problems such as coronary artery disease.

Nuclear Stress Examination

A nuclear stress test is an imaging examination that assesses the blood flow and pumping performance of the heart. A little quantity of radioactive material is injected into the circulation, where it goes to the heart. The heart is then photographed using a specific camera when the patient is at rest and after physical exercise. The test aids in the detection of regions of the heart with restricted blood flow, which indicates coronary artery disease.

Catheterization of the Heart

Cardiac catheterization is an invasive procedure in which a tiny tube called a catheter is inserted into a blood artery in the arm, neck, or groin. The catheter is then advanced to the heart, where a dye is given to aid in the visualization of the blood arteries. The test is used to identify and treat cardiovascular diseases such as coronary artery disease, heart valve issues, and congenital heart abnormalities.

Angiography of the Coronary Artery
A coronary angiography is a form of cardiac catheterization in which the blood arteries around the heart are examined. A dye is administered via the catheter, and X-ray pictures are acquired to assess the function of the coronary arteries and find obstructions.

Angiography via CT
CTA (computed tomography angiography) is a non-invasive imaging technique that employs X-rays to make detailed pictures of the blood arteries in the heart. The test may identify coronary artery disease, aneurysms, and other cardiac problems.

Magnetic Resonance Imaging.
Magnetic resonance imaging (MRI) is a non-invasive imaging procedure that creates comprehensive pictures of the heart's structure

and function using strong magnets and radio waves. The exam may reveal heart anomalies such as congenital heart disease, heart valve issues, and cardiac malignancies.

Blood Examinations

Blood tests may aid in the diagnosis of heart disease by assessing cholesterol levels, blood sugar levels, and other risk factors. High LDL cholesterol levels, for example, are linked to an increased risk of coronary heart disease.

Heart Disease Medical and Surgical Treatments

Heart disease is a critical, sometimes fatal ailment that needs immediate diagnosis and treatment. There are several medicinal and surgical therapies available for heart disease, each suited to the patient's requirements.

Heart Disease Medical Treatments:

Medications

The most frequent therapy for heart disease is medication. They are used to treat symptoms, minimize the risk of complications, and enhance the overall quality of life. The sort of medicine administered will be determined by the precise type of heart disease and the patient's unique requirements. Among the most regularly given drugs are:

ACE inhibitors: These drugs assist to control blood pressure and lessen the chance of having a heart attack or stroke.
Beta-blockers: These drugs assist to minimize the burden on the heart by slowing the heart rate.
Calcium channel blockers: These drugs relax the blood arteries and lower blood pressure.
Diuretics: These drugs assist to decrease the quantity of fluid in the body, which may lower blood pressure and relieve the burden on the heart.
Statins are drugs that help control cholesterol and lessen the risk of heart attack and stroke.

Surgical Heart Disease Treatments:

CABG stands for Coronary Artery Bypass Grafting.
CABG is a surgical treatment used to repair coronary artery blockages. A surgeon will utilize

a healthy blood vessel from another area of the body, such as the leg, to bypass the blocked artery during the treatment. This permits blood to flow freely to the heart muscle, which may alleviate symptoms and lower the risk of problems.

Stenting and Angioplasty
Angioplasty and stenting are minimally invasive treatments used to treat coronary artery blockages. A small tube is introduced into the blocked artery during the treatment, and a balloon is inflated to unblock the artery. To maintain the artery open, a stent may be implanted. This may assist to alleviate symptoms and lower the likelihood of problems.

Repair or replacement of a heart valve
A surgical treatment used to treat damaged or diseased heart valves is heart valve repair or replacement. During the surgery, a surgeon will either repair or replace the damaged valve with a prosthetic valve. This may assist in improving cardiac function and lowering the risk of problems.

Implantable Technology

Certain forms of cardiac disease are treated using implantable devices such as pacemakers and defibrillators. Pacemakers are used to control the cardiac rhythm, while defibrillators are used to treat potentially fatal arrhythmias. These devices may aid in the improvement of cardiac function and the reduction of problems.

Transplantation of the Heart

Heart transplantation is a medical operation in which a damaged heart is removed and replaced with a healthy heart from a donor. It is normally reserved for individuals with end-stage heart failure who have failed all previous medicinal and surgical therapies.

Changes in Lifestyle to Manage Heart Disease

Making lifestyle modifications is an essential part of heart disease management. These modifications may help lower the risk of future heart issues and enhance overall health. Some of the most important lifestyle adjustments that may be done are as follows:

Tobacco use is a significant risk factor for heart disease. Tobacco smoke contains compounds that harm the heart and blood vessels, causing plaque accumulation in the arteries. Quitting smoking may improve your heart health and lower your risk of future heart issues.

Maintain a Healthy Diet: Maintaining a healthy diet is essential for controlling heart disease. A diet low in saturated and trans fats, cholesterol, and salt and rich in fruits, vegetables, whole grains, lean proteins, and healthy fats is suggested. A certified dietician may assist in the development of a tailored nutrition plan.

Maintain a Healthy Weight: Excess weight puts additional pressure on the heart and raises the risk of heart disease. Losing weight and keeping it off may assist improve heart health.

Exercise regularly: Physical exercise is essential for heart health. At least 150 minutes of moderate-intensity aerobic activity or 75 minutes of vigorous-intensity aerobic exercise each week is advised. Resistance exercise and stretching might also help.

Manage Stress: Because stress may lead to heart disease, stress management is an essential element of heart health management. Meditation, deep breathing, and yoga may all be beneficial.

Limit Alcohol use: Excessive alcohol use might raise blood pressure and lead to heart disease. Alcohol intake should be limited to one drink per day for women and two drinks per day for males.

Chronic diseases such as high blood pressure, high cholesterol, and diabetes may all raise the risk of heart disease. These disorders must be managed by medicine, frequent check-ups with a healthcare practitioner, and lifestyle adjustments.

Get adequate Sleep: Because lack of sleep may lead to heart disease, obtaining adequate sleep is critical for heart health. It is advised to get 7-9 hours of sleep every night.

Chapter Eight:

Holistic Therapies to Promote Cardiovascular Health

Cardiovascular disease is a primary cause of mortality globally and encompasses illnesses such as coronary artery disease, heart failure, and stroke. While medical treatments such as drugs and surgical procedures are often required, adopting holistic therapies may also help to maintain cardiovascular health. These treatments target the underlying emotional, mental, and spiritual health issues that might contribute to the development and progression of cardiovascular disease. Here are some natural remedies that may help with cardiovascular health.

Mind-body techniques like meditation, yoga, and tai chi may help decrease stress, anxiety, and depression, all of which are risk factors for cardiovascular disease. These techniques also help with relaxation, sleep quality, and general well-being. Regular meditation has been found in studies to improve blood pressure, decrease inflammation, and minimize the risk of heart disease.

Acupuncture is an ancient Chinese treatment in which small needles are inserted into particular places on the body to enhance energy flow and aid healing. Acupuncture has been found in studies to help decrease blood pressure, lower cholesterol levels, and enhance circulation, all of which may assist cardiovascular health.

Massage treatment may help relieve stress and increase relaxation, both of which can lower blood pressure and heart rate. Massage may also help with cardiovascular health by improving circulation, reducing muscular tension, and relieving discomfort. Furthermore, research has shown that frequent massage helps lower anxiety and sadness, both of which are risk factors for heart disease.

Nutritional counseling: Maintaining cardiovascular health requires a balanced diet, and working with a nutritionist or dietitian may assist ensure that you are receiving the nutrients your body requires. A nutritionist can assist you in developing a customized nutrition plan that is specific to your requirements and tastes. They may also educate and encourage you in making better food choices and developing healthy eating habits.

Certain herbs and supplements may help with cardiovascular health. Garlic, for example, has been demonstrated to decrease cholesterol and blood pressure, while omega-3 fatty acids found in fish oil may help reduce inflammation and improve circulation. Hawthorn, ginger, turmeric, and ginseng are among more herbs that may be beneficial to cardiovascular health.

Physical exercise: Physical activity regularly is vital for cardiovascular health. Exercise may help decrease blood pressure, cholesterol levels, and inflammation. It may also aid in the maintenance of a healthy weight as well as the reduction of stress, anxiety, and sadness. Exercise does not have to be a marathon to be beneficial; even modest activities such as walking, cycling, or swimming may enhance cardiovascular health.

Stress management: Stress is a key risk factor for cardiovascular disease, and stress management is critical for cardiovascular health. Mindfulness meditation, yoga, and tai chi are examples of holistic treatments that may help decrease stress and increase relaxation. Deep breathing exercises, gradual muscle relaxation, and guided visualization are among more stress-reduction approaches.

Sleep hygiene is crucial for cardiovascular health since lack of sleep has been related to an increased risk of heart disease, stroke, and other cardiovascular disorders. Good sleep hygiene, such as avoiding coffee and alcohol before bedtime, sticking to a regular sleep schedule, and providing a pleasant sleep environment, may promote restful sleep and improve cardiovascular health.

Heart Health Herbal Medicine

For decades, herbal therapy has been used to treat a variety of diseases, including heart disease. Many herbs include natural anti-inflammatory and antioxidant characteristics that may benefit cardiovascular health. Here are some herbs that are often used for heart health:

Hawthorn is a popular plant used to treat heart problems. It includes chemicals that may aid in the dilation of blood vessels, the reduction of blood pressure, and the improvement of blood flow to the heart. It may also aid in the reduction of cholesterol and the prevention of blood clots.

Garlic is well-known for its heart-healthy qualities. It may help decrease cholesterol, regulate blood pressure, and prevent blood clots from forming. Garlic may also aid in the improvement of blood flow to the heart and the reduction of inflammation.

Ginger is an anti-inflammatory plant that may assist enhance cardiovascular health. It may assist to decrease inflammation, controlling blood pressure, and preventing blood clot formation.

Turmeric includes curcumin, a substance with potent anti-inflammatory and antioxidant effects. It may aid in the reduction of inflammation, the reduction of cholesterol levels, and the improvement of cardiovascular health.

Ginkgo Biloba is a plant that is often used to boost cognitive performance, but it may also benefit heart health. It may help to increase blood flow to the heart, decrease inflammation, and prevent blood clots from forming.

Green Tea: Green tea includes catechins, which are potent antioxidants that may help enhance cardiovascular health. It may aid in the reduction of inflammation, the reduction of cholesterol levels, and the improvement of blood flow to the heart.

Cayenne pepper includes a chemical known as capsaicin, which may assist enhance cardiovascular health. It may aid in the reduction of inflammation, the reduction of blood pressure, and the improvement of blood flow to the heart.

It is important to remember that herbal medicine should only be taken with caution and under the supervision of a healthcare expert. Some herbs may interact with drugs and are thus not suitable for everyone.

Cardiovascular Health Supplements

Supplements may complement a balanced diet and lifestyle to help protect cardiovascular health. It is crucial to remember, however, that supplements should not be taken in place of medicine recommended by a healthcare practitioner.

Here are some supplements that have been examined for their possible cardiovascular health benefits:

Omega-3 Fatty Acids: Omega-3 fatty acids contain anti-inflammatory effects and may help decrease triglyceride levels, blood pressure, and the risk of heart disease. If you don't get enough omega-3 fatty fish in your diet, the American Heart Association suggests taking an omega-3 supplement.

Coenzyme Q10 (CoQ10): CoQ10 is a natural antioxidant that aids in the production of energy in cells. It has been demonstrated to offer potential heart health advantages such as enhancing endothelial function and lowering inflammation. Some research suggests that taking CoQ10 supplements may help with heart failure symptoms.

Magnesium: Magnesium is an essential element for general health and has been found to offer possible cardiovascular health advantages such as decreasing blood pressure and lowering the risk of heart disease. It may be found in a variety of complete foods, including leafy greens, nuts, and whole grains, although supplementation may be essential for those with low levels.

Vitamin D: Vitamin D is vital for bone health and may potentially have cardiovascular advantages, such as lowering inflammation and increasing endothelial function. It may be gained by sunshine and meals such as fatty fish and fortified dairy products, although supplements may be required for those with low levels.

Red Yeast Rice: Red yeast rice is a traditional Chinese medicine prepared from fermented rice. It includes monacolin K, a substance that has been demonstrated to decrease cholesterol levels. It should be noted, however, that certain red yeast rice supplements may contain high quantities of monacolin K, which might have adverse effects comparable to statins.

Chapter Nine:

The Importance of Mindset in Cardiovascular Health

The significance of attitude in heart health is becoming more relevant as research suggests that one's psychological state may have a substantial influence on one's cardiovascular health. In this chapter, we will look at the connection between mentality and heart health and provide advice on how to cultivate a good mindset for optimum cardiovascular health.

Heart Health and Mindset

The relationship between mentality and heart health is gaining attention in the field of cardiology. A positive outlook has been demonstrated in studies to reduce the risk of heart disease and improve results for people who have already been diagnosed with heart disease.

According to research, those who have a happy view of life are less likely to get heart disease. According to research published in the European Heart Journal, those who have an optimistic view had a 30% reduced chance of acquiring heart disease than those who have a negative outlook. Another research published in the American Journal of Cardiology discovered that persons who had a happy attitude had a decreased chance of dying from heart disease.

A positive outlook may benefit persons who currently have heart disease in addition to lowering their chance of developing it. People who have a happy view of life are more likely to participate in healthy habits such as regular exercise and a nutritious diet, which may help them manage their heart disease and avoid future issues, according to research.

Importance of Positive Psychology in Cardiovascular health

The scientific study of the characteristics and virtues that allow people and societies to flourish is referred to as positive psychology. It is a field that promotes well-being, happiness, and pleasant emotions by focusing on the positive elements of the human experience. Positive thinking has been demonstrated in studies to have a major influence on heart health.

According to research, those who have a happy view of life are less likely to get heart disease. A Harvard School of Public Health researcher discovered that those with the greatest levels of optimism had a 50% decreased chance of acquiring cardiovascular disease than those with the lowest levels of optimism. almost the course of 10 years, the researchers monitored almost 70,000 women.

A cheerful attitude might also assist those who already have heart disease manage their condition better. Individuals who are enthusiastic about their abilities to control their disease are more likely to embrace healthy lifestyle modifications such as a nutritious diet, frequent exercise, and quitting smoking, according to research. These modifications may assist to enhance heart health and lower the chance of future issues.

A cheerful attitude may also help to minimize stress and worry, both of which are established risk factors for heart disease. Chronic stress may cause the production of chemicals that raise heart rate and blood pressure, causing artery damage and increasing the risk of heart disease. A cheerful attitude may help people manage stress and lower their chance of getting heart disease.

Positive Mindset Cultivation Techniques

Here are some suggestions for creating a happy mentality to improve cardiovascular health:

Gratitude is a very effective strategy for creating a happy mentality. Taking time to reflect on what you are thankful for regularly may help you change your emphasis on the good elements of life, lowering stress and creating a feeling of well-being.

Mindfulness is the discipline of being present in the present moment and noticing one's thoughts and sensations without judgment. Regular mindfulness practice has been demonstrated to decrease blood pressure, reduce stress, and increase general well-being.

Maintain social connections: Social connection is a vital part of both mental and physical wellness. Keeping in touch with family, friends, and the community may give a feeling of belonging and support, lowering stress and boosting general well-being.

Setting realistic objectives may create a feeling of purpose and drive, creating a good mentality. To establish a feeling of achievement and momentum, start small and build on your triumphs.

Positive self-talk is important since it has a big influence on our thinking and general well-being. Practice speaking to yourself in a positive and supportive tone, emphasizing your successes and talents.

Activities that you like may bring a feeling of pleasure and fulfillment, lowering stress and increasing general well-being. Make time for your favorite hobbies and pastimes.
Seek help when needed: Recognize when you need help and seek out loved ones or a mental health expert for assistance. Seeking assistance when you need it may help you minimize stress and improve your overall well-being.

Conclusion

Finally, heart disease is preventable and controllable with a comprehensive approach to cardiovascular health. You can minimize your risk of heart disease by integrating lifestyle changes such as regular exercise, a good diet, stress management, and eliminating dangerous behaviors such as smoking.

Acupuncture, meditation, and herbal medicine are all holistic therapies that may help with cardiovascular health and complement traditional therapy.

Furthermore, mentality and positive psychology are important in supporting heart health and lowering the risk of repeated cardiac episodes. You can take charge of your well-being and live a better, happier life by taking a proactive approach to your heart health.

Remember that prevention is vital, and even minor adjustments may have a big effect on lowering your risk of heart disease. You can

fight heart disease and enjoy a long, healthy life
if you work hard enough.